The MindBody Workbook

Volume Two

Thirty Days of Guided Journaling and Affirmations
for Chronic Pain, Stress, and Other Disorders

David Schechter, M.D.
with
Justin Barker, Psy.D.

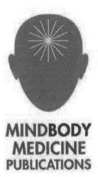

MINDBODY MEDICINE PUBLICATIONS

© 2023 MindBody Medicine Publications
All rights reserved.

Research supports the use of expressive writing for a variety of health conditions. Individuals with irritable bowel syndrome, fibromyalgia, tension headaches, TMJ, chronic fatigue, anxiety, and some auto-immune conditions may also benefit greatly.

The MindBody Workbook
Volume Two

**Thirty Days of Guided Journaling and Affirmations
for Chronic Pain, Stress, and Other Disorders**

Published by: MindBody Medicine Publications
               10811 Washington Blvd, Suite 250
               Culver City, CA 90232   www.MindBodyMedicine.com

All rights reserved by the publisher.
No part of this book may be reproduced or transmitted in any form or by any means including electronic, mechanical, photocopying, recording, or information storage system without written permission from the author/publisher, except for the inclusion of brief quotations in a review.

Printed in the United States of America

Schechter, David. Barker, Justin.
    MindBody Workbook Volume Two/David Schechter, MD. Justin Barker, Psy.D.
    Includes bibliographical references and index
    ISBN: 978-1-929997-00-8

©MindBody Medicine Publications

First Published   March 2023

Warning—Disclaimer
Anyone using this book for a medical condition should be under the care of a physician. The reader and his/her physician should decide appropriate use of this book in conjunction with usual and customary medical techniques and treatments. The reader should have appropriate medical examinations to diagnose his/her condition and exclude serious illnesses that may require immediate or aggressive treatment.

Dedications and Acknowledgments

We dedicate this Workbook to John E. Sarno, M.D. who cured my (DS) knee pain decades ago and my (JB) back pain and taught us both about TMS, his novel and important diagnosis for much chronic pain (and other conditions). Dr. Sarno was a true pioneer in medicine and died in 2017 after a long life and productive career. We remember the 100th anniversary of his birth in 2023.

DS: And to my wife, Lisa for being a helpmate and my longtime partner, as well as a precise editor when called upon. To my sons Aidan and Noah for keeping me humble...very, very humble.

JB: To my wife, Christa, for always believing in me and showing me what it means to truly play.

Most of all, we dedicate this workbook to all of the patients who courageously break out of the model of pain management and consider that true healing is possible. Your willingness to learn about the mindbody connection, work on your emotions, improve your wellbeing, and remain convinced that your life can change and you can heal from pain is a true inspiration.

Table of Contents

Dedications and Acknowledgments	iii
Introduction	vii
What is TMS? A Quick Review	1
How to Use this Workbook to Heal	3
Ideally, Get a TMS Diagnosis	6
Your Complete TMS Healing Program	7
What Do I Need to Do to Heal? Quick Reference Sheet	11
Our Personal Experiences with TMS Pain	12
Familiarizing Yourself with the Resources at the End of this Workbook	18
Volume Two	19
Day Zero	21
Day "Double Zero"	29
Week One	32
Week Two	51
Week Two	66
Week Three	69
Week Four	90
Final Days	105
Final Days	108
Affirmations	111
Afterword and Appendices	113
Ten Reasons You May Be Struggling to Heal	115
Ten Ways To Understand and Overcome the Issues Above	116

Finding a MindBody Practitioner	117
Bonus: Other Approaches to Journaling	119
Bibliography	121
About the Authors	122
The MindBody Healing Journey	124
Other Books by David Schechter, M.D.	127

Introduction

Why another MindBody Workbook? Since I (DS) wrote the first MindBody Workbook in 1999, there have been almost a dozen books written about the Tension Myoneural Syndrome (TMS) approach to pain and other disorders including *Think Away Your* Pain, published in 2014. Aren't there enough books on the MindBody connection?

The original MindBody Workbook remains popular and important in that its design guides the interested and motivated individual to **make** the mindbody connection, not just read about it. The format is a structured or "guided" journal that takes about thirty days to complete. Journaling, or expressive writing as it is sometimes called, has been a highly successful and significant component of my clinical practice in treating individuals with TMS and related conditions for over twenty-five years.

Justin Barker Psy.D. (JB) and I wrote this second Volume because readers have requested an updated perspective, another month of guided journaling, and because so much more has been learned about the significance of expressive writing. In addition, we have many more years of experience working with patients with TMS and more knowledge of the right prompts to help people identify key feelings and life experiences that can help those seeking relief from pain, stress, and other conditions.

This Workbook also works well with *Think Away Your Pain* and *The MindBody Healing Journey* online course. We are including detailed tips for healing, focusing on self-talk strategies, affirmations, and other day-to-day approaches to make the changes in your brain that are essential for the pain to go away. There is a unique affirmation for each day of the Workbook and it is typically selected to connect to the topic of the day or week.

Because of the importance of building confidence in and accepting the diagnosis in order to heal, we have also added weekly reminders to look at the evidence supporting your diagnosis of TMS and to confront your doubts. Methodically identifying barriers to accepting the diagnosis can be instrumental in getting the pain to go away.

Some of you have completed the original thirty-day Workbook. For others, this is the first time you have done journaling in this context. The prompts will be applicable for both groups and I want to commend you for embarking on your healing journey.

David Schechter, M.D.

What is TMS?
A Quick Review

Many of you using this Workbook will already have some familiarity with TMS from reading one of Dr. Sarno's, Dr. Schechter's, or other TMS books; through an app, or through a medical visit with a TMS practitioner. However, for some of you this may be the first time you are really encountering this information, so we have included a brief review of TMS. Even if you are already familiar with TMS, it can be useful to have a concise explanation to refer back to.

Tension Myoneural Syndrome (TMS) is a term coined by Dr. John Sarno to describe persistent pain and other bodily (or somatic) sensations that are not primarily caused by a structural or biochemical issue in the body. Instead, the cause is related to the mind/brain. Simply put, it's more about psychology than peripheral biomechanics or a disease. Many people with TMS have either tried structural approaches (injections, physical therapy, acupuncture, chiropractic or even surgery) with limited or no success, or have been told by a medical professional(s) that they can't find anything wrong.

We call this category of conditions psychophysiologic or psychosomatic or mindbody because the connection between the central nervous system (mind/brain and emotions) and the rest of the human body is the key to diagnosis and treatment. Other names for this disorder include PPD PsychoPhysiologic Disorder (PPD), neuroplastic pain, nociplastic pain, central pain sensitization, and Mind Body Syndrome.

Psychologically speaking, Dr. Sarno hypothesized that physical symptoms such as pain were a way to distract the mind from repressed emotions that would feel threatening. In other words, if someone feels angry but also believes that anger is "bad" or "wrong," the mind might try to distract the person from this feeling by creating pain or excessively focusing on existing sensations. Dr. Sarno focused mostly on repressed anger or rage as the key underlying emotion.

Building upon his work, we have learned that there are many more emotions that can feel threatening for people to experience. Some people with TMS have strong feelings of guilt, shame, anger, sadness, grief, fear, anxiety, or other feelings underlying the persistent symptoms. People with TMS also tend to have similar personality characteristics, codified as Type T, including high degrees of self-criticism, internal pressure, perfectionism, and ultra-high standards for the world.

An important fact to understand is that there can be structural variations in the body not causing the symptom. Research has repeatedly demonstrated that even if medical imaging finds a minor "abnormality," this does not necessarily cause pain. The classic example of this is that many people with disc bulges have no pain. One way to think about it is that different parts of our bodies go through changes akin to how hair goes gray (we sometimes call it "gray hairs of the spine"). So your body is typically fine, which is great news!

What hundreds of thousands of people have experienced, including both of us, is that once you understand that nothing is structurally wrong with the body, this can bring a feeling of relief and sometimes full healing. However, often one needs to both understand this point (education helps), and also engage in psychological and emotional reflection to identify important feelings that are needing expression (this is where journaling in this Workbook or psychotherapy helps).

So, to summarize: TMS is all about understanding that your body is basically fine. You are healthy, resilient, safe, and can heal. That is what bodies do naturally – they heal! The pain is related to paying too much attention to a specific body area or sensation and having too much fear about what might be wrong and whether it's permanent. The pain may also be serving as a distraction from unpleasant or threatening feelings which need to be explored.

(For a more comprehensive review of TMS, see *Think Away Your Pain*.)

How to Use this Workbook to Heal

The purpose of this Workbook is to help you uncover and connect to the specific emotional issues that may be inhibiting your healing. In our combined nearly fifty years in medical training, practice, and psychological training and psychotherapy, we can attest to the powerful effect of utilizing the mindbody connection to heal patients and even ourselves. Focusing on emotions as a path to healing can feel strange at first, but we have seen it work over many decades. Moreover, gaining better emotional awareness and insight has many benefits beyond just healing from physical pain!

During the month of this program, the active user of this workbook will respond to questions and prompts that we have found useful with many of our patients. Gradually or sometimes suddenly, the user will gain insight and awareness into the role that emotions may be playing in their illness or condition. The writing also alleviates and releases some of the emotional tension that has been misdirected toward the creation or amplification of physical symptoms.

The time required is not extensive, just ten to twenty minutes a day. Keep in mind that more is not always better with TMS; focusing too much on healing can become another distraction from living your life. However, commitment and accountability is essential to achieve the maximal benefit from this thirty-day program. The user does not have to write every day, but it is better to make that a goal and still be satisfied and proud if you write five or six days each week of the program.

Even if your pain or health condition originated with a physical injury or a structural or biochemical abnormality, if it persists despite appropriate treatment, the mental and emotional aspects may be significant in making your symptoms worse, and therefore this workbook is often helpful in these cases as well. Research (see *Think Away Your Pain* for details) has demonstrated that chronic pain actually resides in a different part of the brain than acute pain and that this part is more connected to human emotion!

This Workbook may be used independently or in combination with the medical treatment program developed by your treating doctor. We hope that many more primary care and specialty physicians who treat chronic pain, irritable bowel syndrome (IBS), temporomandibular joint dysfunction (TMJ), chronic fatigue, anxiety, and some other conditions will see fit to recommend journaling/expressive writing to their patients. Psychologists can utilize the Workbook as an adjunct to therapy, either individual or group therapy. Therapy is typically once a week. This Workbook can fill in the gap between therapy sessions. The material written during these days may make therapy more useful, focused, and even faster. The Workbook can stimulate emotional connections and memories that can be analyzed further in therapy sessions.

In our experience, it is the act of answering these questions, writing, and making associations and connections that is crucial to recovery. Some may choose to type their answers on a computer, although freehand writing may have some advantages in terms of accessing the brain in a different way than typing does (see "Journaling by Hand vs. Computer" at http://bit.ly/HandJrnl). Recording your spoken answers on an electronic device can be effective as well. Ultimately, though, we believe handwriting is the ideal choice based upon experience and current research.

This process of self-examination and re-programming the nervous system out of the vicious cycle of worry, fear, anger, and pain can take some time and some effort. The questions in this book and in the original Workbook are designed to enable expression of important feelings and the making of connections and associations between past experiences and present discomforts.

If you write some particularly nasty stuff and are concerned someone may find the Workbook, it is permissible to rip that page out, tear it up, and throw it away. Sometimes this can be therapeutic in and of itself. The "write and rip" approach is sometimes called negative writing.

In this Workbook we also include pages that focus more on positive emotions such as gratitude and liking oneself. We have learned over the years in dealing with thousands of "Type T" personality TMS patients (those individuals who are predisposed to chronic pain, etc.) that too much negative expression can feel emotionally defeating to some. So, we have gradually started adding these pages over the years to balance that off. These positive expression days will be helpful for anyone which is why they are included every week.

As a final note, many people with TMS have perfectionistic tendencies and/or a strong desire to do things "right." Sometimes this can make journaling feel difficult, and we hear people express worry about if they are journaling in the right way; accessing enough feelings through journaling; or another related concern. If you use this workbook and answer the questions as best as you can, you are doing it right! We have purposefully avoided providing examples of journaling entries because we want each user to approach the journal with your own words and we trust that if you complete this workbook and answer all of the questions, it will help your pain.

The MindBody Workbook and The MindBody Healing Journey Course

In addition to this Workbook and Volume One of the Workbook, we have created an online course called The MindBody Healing Journey. Each of these materials evolved naturally out of the clinical work. We know the benefits of home education and practice to supplement the office diagnosis. There has also been increased interest throughout the world in the TMS work and we hope that MindBody healing approaches will be increasingly used. As TMS information has proliferated, we have also seen an increased need for a systematic approach that does not overwhelm people with different techniques, tools, strategies, and skills.

The process of healing from a mindbody disorder is variable. For some people, just getting an office diagnosis is sufficient to initiate a big change. For others, reading a book helps to tip the scale toward healing. Many individuals require a more systematic and extensive process. This Workbook and our treatment program in its entirety form a supportive system (MD office consultation, follow-up visits in office or via videoconference, journaling, and sometimes working with a psychotherapist). This Workbook fosters a disciplined, structured approach to working through your pain problem and changing your thinking process. However, if you find that you want more information about TMS, more information about how to work with and process emotions, or more information about frequently asked questions and barriers, the video course is a useful supplement. You can find more information at https://www.mindbodymedicine.com/online-course

Ideally, Get a TMS Diagnosis

We recommend a formal medical examination prior to utilizing this Workbook. Even if you are fairly confident that you have TMS, what we consistently find is that a formal medical examination by a TMS trained physician can create a significant confidence boost and expedite healing. We suggest that you seek out a TMS physician—one who is available nearby, or via telemedicine.

A good primary care physician or an appropriate subspecialist in your area can also help you exclude serious or life-threatening causes of back and neck pain such as tumors, fractures, rheumatoid arthritis, or even cancer. If your doctor supports a conservative (i.e. a non-surgical approach to your problem), even if that doctor is not familiar with mindbody medicine or TMS, you can appropriately use this Workbook as part of your treatment program. You can also confidently use this Workbook if you have been told by medical professionals that they can't find anything wrong or that your medical symptom(s) is not well understood by the medical community.

It is our hope that in the not-too-distant future that this Workbook and similar materials will be routinely recommended by many practitioners of different medical and alternative specialties for their patients with chronic pain, mindbody, and stress related disorders. The recognition and acknowledgment of mindbody disorders in the medical field would alleviate a great deal of suffering.

In the meantime, this Workbook, *Think Away Your Pain*, and other books and materials, some described on Dr. Schechter's web site www.mindbodymedicine.com and others in the Bibliography, are available for someone actively exploring and seeking a mindbody approach to healing. The first web page of the website listed has links to podcasts and other free recordings.

More scientific evidence for this treatment approach is presented in Chapter VI of Dr. Schechter's book *Think Away Your Pain*. For more information about how to find a mindbody practitioner see "Finding a MindBody Practitioner" at the end of this Workbook.

Your Complete TMS Healing Program

We are going to outline and explain all of the essential elements of your healing program. Key elements are: develop the knowledge of TMS needed to understand that nothing is structurally wrong; accept the diagnosis; journal and use affirmations; resume physical activity; and express your emotions.

Knowledge and Acceptance

1) Read and re-read books on this subject, ideally more than one. As we have explained, this workbook is a companion guide to Dr. Schechter's book, *Think Away Your Pain*. But in addition to that book, other great choices are in the bibliography of this workbook. If you do not choose to read *Think Away Your Pain*, this Workbook can still be incredibly powerful and important.

2) Expose yourself consistently to other materials in the TMS universe. We include a list of online resources in the bibliography and on the first page of Dr. Schechter's website, www.mindbodymedicine.com, in a box in the middle of the page titled *Media/Education*. We have listed updated links to various podcasts, radio, and TV interviews that we have done. These will provide more information about TMS and will counteract the incessant chatter you may find in the media and online discussions about surgery and other procedures for your pain that you might not need and that can be counterproductive to your healing.

3) Consider the *The MindBody Healing Journey* online course. If you do the course, stick to perhaps thirty minutes a night. Some patients study thirty minutes of the course every other day and complete the course in ten days. The course also includes even

shorter segments. Focus on letting the information sink in on a deeper and more emotional level instead of focusing on trying to get through the course as quickly as possible.

4) Increase your confidence in your TMS healing journey. Doubt is a huge impediment to success and pain recovery, so we've included an Evidence Sheet for each week of the workbook to help you become more confident in your diagnosis and approach. It is very important that you systematically work on addressing your doubt about the diagnosis and about your ability to heal. The Evidence Sheet has room to both list the doubts and also generate solutions to overcome doubts.

Journal, Affirmations, and Emotional Expression

1) Journal for 10 to 15 minutes a day, maybe 20 if you write a lot or write slowly. Be open with your feelings, look inside, look to the past, and accept your emotions. Express yourself and try to understand some of the pressures and stressors in your life. Be forgiving and self-compassionate even as you are being truly honest and authentic.

2) Positive Self-Talk: self-talk is an amazing tool to help with reprogramming the brain away from pain. Dr. Sarno used the term "affirmations" and we use both "affirmations" and "positive self-talk."

    Three examples are:

    I am going to be fine. There is nothing seriously wrong. I am healthy.
    I am strong. My back is healthy. I will be active and free.
    The pain is TMS. It is from stress and I am learning to deal with it.

    Try writing another five to ten personalized self-talk messages. Repeat one of the messages above, or one from the ThinkUp app (see below) list, or your own message. This takes ten to thirty seconds each time. Try doing it several times an hour when you remember.

3) Visualization: We find that following self-talk with visualizing an image that makes you feel peaceful and calm (e.g. sunset, beach, mountain, forest) for another ten or twenty seconds or longer is a great way to lower the tension in your nervous system in a slightly different way. Experiment with visualizations to enhance your self-talk and ability to calm yourself.

4) Affirmation Apps: Another great resource for affirmations is the ThinkUp app. You can download ThinkUp to your smartphone or tablet for a free trial from the App Store or at (https://apple.co/2XoCeRC). Under the category: authors/experts, you will find Dr. Schechter's list of 16 affirmations for pain. An interesting element of the ThinkUp app is that you can record your affirmations in your own voice for playback once or twice a day or as needed. There are premium features, as usual, for a fee.

Resuming Physical Activity

Try to gradually be more active if you have restricted yourself due to your symptoms. Note that being more active is not just about physical exercise; it's about resuming the activities you did prior to TMS. For someone with back pain, this might mean resuming physical exercise. For someone with IBS, this might mean eating a previously feared food. For someone with headaches, this might mean attending a social engagement for multiple hours. The point is you begin living your life as you did prior to TMS. Increasing your physical activity will reinforce to your mind that your body is healthy and your condition is improving. Moving every day and in different ways is important. Eventually doing the activities that you have feared returning to is an important part of mid-late stage healing.

How long does it take to heal?

The simple answer is it takes as long as it takes.

The longer answer is that if you have had a diagnosis made of TMS by a doctor, or you are personally cleared from any other diagnoses and are deep into acceptance of this TMS diagnosis, you should make some improvement in three to four weeks and more improvement each month that follows. There can be steps backward along the way, unfortunately. Everyone is different and every case is different. For some, the healing process may be much longer and that is common; this is not something of which to feel ashamed.

A few people feel amazingly better in a few days. This is not common. If they are better that quickly, they are still subject to Stage six of healing (doubt), and Stage eight (ups and downs of progress and flare-ups). These Healing Stages are described in more detail in *Think Away Your Pain.* The healing journey is not a race. It is a process. **What is critically important is that you do not put pressure on yourself to heal quickly.** Putting pressure on yourself to heal quickly will slow down your healing process, not speed it up.

What Do I Need to Do to Heal? Quick Reference Sheet

Because people so often feel unsure of what to focus on during the healing journey, we have created this one-page Quick Reference Sheet to be photographed or placed in your pocket or bag for easy reference. Use this as a quick reference if you feel stuck and unsure of what you're needing to do to heal. Questions to ask yourself:

1. Am I finding ways to regularly experience and express my emotions, including ones that are less comfortable?
2. Am I regularly listening to, reading, and learning about TMS and the mindbody connection so that I am confident in both the diagnosis of TMS and also my ability to heal from it?
3. Am I resuming physical activities and any other activities that I was avoiding because of the pain or other TMS sensations? If I am still too afraid to engage in certain activities, do I have a plan about how I will get closer and closer to engaging in those activities?
4. Am I finding ways to de-stress and be kinder to myself?
5. Am I finding ways to have fun and play? (Remember that when you are involved in play, you are much less likely to think about pain which is why this is so important.)
6. Am I finding ways to address any lingering doubts I have? (Remember that it's OK to have doubts, but you should have a plan of how you will address them. If you have doubts that persist, a professional consultation is usually a good idea.)

If at any point you feel stuck in your healing journey, you can also reference our **Top 10 Reasons You are Struggling to Heal** at the end of this Workbook.

Our Personal Experiences with TMS Pain

Dr. Schechter's Story

My first exposure to clinical mindbody medicine was when I was diagnosed by Dr. Sarno as having Tension Myositis Syndrome, later Tension Myoneural Syndrome (or TMS), while a freshman medical student at New York University in 1981. I had been suffering from severe knee pain, worse with running and basketball, for some time. During my first year in medical school, the knee pain became severe enough that I was forced to curtail these two recreational activities. When I did so, my knee pain got a little better, but any attempt to return to sports made it worse again. TMS is a diagnosis that connects physical symptoms with a mind/brain or mindbody/emotional cause for the symptoms.

I sought treatment at the medical school's student health department and was even referred to a Professor of Orthopedics, a knee specialist, and one of the New York Yankees' team physicians. He prescribed anti-inflammatory medication and an exercise program. I diligently performed these exercises and strengthened the muscles around my knees. Despite this added strength, I still had pain with any significant athletic activity.

The next step back then was the arthrogram, an x-ray test that involves the injection of a dye-containing solution into the knee joint. Yes, this was as painful as it sounds, especially when performed by a resident in radiology learning the procedure on my knees while his professor supervised him. The results were negative for any tear that would require surgery. They showed a "normal variant" appearance to my meniscal cartilage, which the orthopedic professor felt was not significant. I was advised to keep doing my exercises and that surgery was not likely to be helpful in my case. MRI imaging was not used commonly for this for a few more years, unfortunately.

My diagnosis was tendonitis, aka "runner's knee." I sought out the advice of John E. Sarno,

M.D., Professor of Rehabilitation Medicine at NYU. He had lectured to my class in anatomy during our first semester in school on the musculoskeletal system. He seemed a logical choice for recommendations about exercise or other rehabilitative techniques to help my knee recover.

The advice Dr. Sarno gave me when I entered his office was surprising and ultimately career-defining for me. After a very brief discussion of my symptoms and normal test results, he told me that, in his experience, 95% of these chronic pain syndromes were "tension related." Stunned at this unexpected twist, I responded that I had heard of migraine headaches being due to stress, but knee pain from basketball? His response was to invite me to his evening lecture on this subject that he gave to his patients. He told me I could come in for a more detailed consultation after that seminar if I wished.

I attended the presentation with more than a little skepticism, but with a lot of interest. I had gradually become aware of the fact that I was prone to physical ailments related to stress. I had some irritable bowel symptoms during my teenage years and I associated them with anxiety-provoking social events.

Athletic competitions during college tended to provoke the same kinds of symptoms. When I was a teenager, my family doctor had mentioned stress in response to a couple of my minor illnesses, but I wasn't yet sure that he was right. I wasn't yet able to accept his diagnosis.

Dr. Sarno's evening lecture was attended by about twenty or thirty individuals, all older than my 21 years, some considerably so. They seemed like a group of normal, superficially successful, well-adjusted people. The lecture began with a discussion of anatomy and worked its way through psychology and a description of the Tension Myositis Syndrome, as Dr. Sarno called it then. Most of the discussion focused on back pain, but he mentioned that it was applicable to other painful conditions and a variety of psychosomatic disorders. Specifically, he mentioned irritable bowel syndrome, allergies, asthma, and migraines.

Gradually, the explanations began not only to make sense to me but explained to me a lot about myself. I noticed my own tendency to worry about my knee pain similar to the case examples that Dr. Sarno presented. I had been reading everything I could find in the medical school library about knee pain and was very focused on cause and cure. My awareness of and focus on structural variations in my legs (tibial torsion, or curved shin bone) and flat feet led to no pain relief, but more worry. I had tried knee braces and arch supports without any change. Also, my past history of tension-related bowel symptoms and prior back spasms in college seemed eerily consistent with the profile of the TMS sufferer which Dr. Sarno described.

The clarity of Dr. Sarno's explanation for my knee pain, "tendonalgia," as he called it, and other conditions, really struck a chord. As I walked home that evening, I felt less worried and more hopeful than I had in quite a while. By the time I arrived home, I was excited, but also very calm. I sat on the edge of my bed and thought about the evening presentation. I could feel my tension level dropping and my knee pain disappearing.

Over the next few days and weeks, my knee pain dissipated. I did see Dr. Sarno in consultation and his examination of my back confirmed that I possessed the characteristic TMS tender points. (see Bibliography for diagrams). I also had the personality traits that are commonly associated with TMS.

I returned to active basketball and running. I occasionally had mild knee discomfort, but nothing like my prior level of symptoms and it didn't stop me from being active in sports. The beneficial effect of return to these beloved pastimes and the stress release from these physical outlets only seemed to create more relaxation and well-being. The negativity and worry about my knee had dissipated. Now, as a born worrier, I could go back to worrying about other things, like medical school and my social life.

The pain had indeed functioned as a distraction for me from dealing with other issues. It also became a hindrance in coping with these issues. As I recovered from the pain, I quickly became a believer and even a proselytizer to the cause of psychosomatic or mindbody medicine. Often this perspective was not well received in a highly traditional and conventional medical school environment among my fellow students and faculty.

The following summer, with the support of a work-study research grant, I performed 177 telephonic interviews under Dr. Sarno's guidance, and the results confirmed the validity of his approach with a large group of former patients. The details of this study are described in at least two of his books (see Bibliography). For me, they provided supporting evidence for my own experience with TMS and a basis for further understanding and treating the disorder.

I completed my medical education and residency training and have been involved in clinical practice, teaching, and medical quality research and review. I have maintained a TMS perspective and approach to treating chronic back pain and other conditions in my training and career.

Not infrequently, I have diagnosed patients as suffering from mindbody disorders including individuals with headaches, pelvic pain, and even eczema. Many of these patients have benefited tremendously from learning about and applying the mindbody connection to their problem.

Beginning in the mid-1990's, I opened a private practice and was fortunate enough to begin to receive a good number of referrals from Dr. Sarno's office in New York. These were individuals who lived on the West Coast and had familiarity with TMS from his books or had friends who were his patients. I began to see more people who were interested and open to utilizing a novel mindbody approach and further developed my ability to treat these conditions. Again and again, I found that educating people about the mindbody connection and teaching them to think psychologically was crucial to their improvement.

During the early years of my private practice, I began to offer the lecture/seminar group class inspired by Dr. Sarno's educational lectures to his patients. Later, I focused more on the initial office consultation combined with the use of home educational materials including an audio-program, later the original *MindBody Workbook*, a DVD called *The MindBody Patient Panel* and my book, *Think Away Your Pain*. Recently I have begun to offer a Zoom group on a weekly basis, leading this group along with Dr. Justin Barker and an online course called *The MindBody Healing Journey*.

Dr. Barker's Story

When I look back on life, I had TMS symptoms since my early teen years when I was diagnosed with chronic knee tendonitis. For many years, I thought that running was hard on the knees and just assumed that any movement not called walking was slowly deteriorating my body. My next symptom was shoulder pain which medical professionals said was due to a "strength imbalance" because of a surgery performed on my right wrist. I was told that everything was "interconnected" which is why a right wrist surgery created pain in my left shoulder.

When I had surgery on my wrist for torn ligaments and a ruptured tendon, the surgeon also informed me that I had loose ligaments and that a normal person would have instead shattered bones in my wrist instead of tearing ligaments. "Loose ligaments" became my go-to explanation for various subsequent pains I experienced.

In my mid-20's, I was deadlifting and felt a sudden pain. I quickly developed the belief that because I was told I was "hypermobile" in my back, I had over-extended my back when deadlifting which caused my injury. My back pain started in my lower back and then developed into pain shooting down my leg as well. Periodically, my upper back would burn, too.

I saw various medical doctors and physical therapists and was told I had a "pinched nerve" albeit with an unremarkable MRI. One physical therapist also informed me that I had scoliosis and should have been put in a back brace when I was a child.

A few people had mentioned John Sarno to me over the years, but I didn't think anything of it. One day, I was doing a physical therapy exercise in which I had a blood pressure cuff beneath my back and was working on minute contractions because the physical therapist thought that a specific sub-region of my abdomen was weak. At that moment, I decided that I had enough. I picked up *Healing Back Pain* and within two months I was pain-free. It felt like a miracle!

Of course that miracle ended and I went back to my Type T personality with a heavy dose of perfectionism, workaholism, anxiety, and stress. Thankfully, knowing about TMS and subsequently dedicating my clinical career to the treatment of TMS, I have successfully healed from: foot pain, knee "tendonitis," groin pain, testicular pain, irritable bowel syndrome, tennis elbow, rotator cuff pain, neck pain, and chronic dry eyes, which a world-class ophthalmologist said would never heal.

I have experienced both the "book cure" by reading Dr. Sarno's book and quickly improving as well as slow, long, and difficult emotional work healing. I had to diligently journal, reduce stress, and examine what was happening emotionally at the time which was leading to a new TMS symptom. In my psychotherapy practice, I have also seen the full range of symptoms and the full range of healing timelines. Sometimes all it takes to improve is a clear belief in TMS and a healing attitude. Sometimes it takes examining traumas, making more significant lifestyle changes, or changing relationships.

What I love about TMS work are the people with TMS. They are some of the most kind, caring, thoughtful, hard-working, and dedicated people I have had the privilege of working with. To examine one's emotional life as a pathway to healing is an immense act of courage. I draw strength from and admire every person on the TMS healing journey.

Underlying Principles: The Twelve Stages of Healing

One Last Pep Talk Before You Journal

Dr. Schechter details in *Think Away Your Pain* the Twelve Stages of Healing from TMS that we believe are commonly seen in the successful patient. We are including five underlying principles of the Twelve Stages and how to apply them because we believe that these principles can serve as your compass for healing. This is especially valuable when you are not sure where to focus your time and attention.

1. **Education**. Dr. Sarno used to say, "education is the penicillin" for TMS. We have also found that education is invaluable. Reading one or more of the books, listening to podcasts or audible books, watching videos are all important elements. Each of you knows how you learn best. See our Bibliography to further explore educational resources.
2. **Confirmation and acceptance of the diagnosis**. Accepting the diagnosis and believing in the method you will need to pursue is essential. The ideal is to see a local TMS physician, but we know that will not be geographically feasible for many of you. You

can get to the point of acceptance without an MD visit, it is just a bit harder. Look closely at the pluses and minuses in your mind of this diagnosis. Do the pluses and the evidence in favor exceed the minuses, lingering questions, and doubts? This is an important step. Be systematic and do your best to get to the point of acceptance. Of course, ensure all serious diagnoses have been excluded.

3. **Shift from physical treatments to mind/brain treatments**. If you already have done a lot of physical therapy, acupuncture, massage, or chiropractic, more is unlikely to fix a persistent pain problem. So, switch your focus, your time and your resources toward fully embracing the TMS treatment model. This may involve ordering some materials, seeing a doctor, or even psychotherapy visits in person or via videoconference. This is the path to success for TMS, so step onto it. Even if a physical treatment gives you temporary relief, such as seeing the chiropractor and then feeling better for a few hours to a day or two, doing physical treatments along with TMS may cause internal conflict or confusion and inhibit healing.

4. **TMS healing is not easy.** Try not to get discouraged. It takes work. Most people do not have an overnight cure. Be persistent, seek support from a physician, therapist, or maybe a friend who has used this approach. Be patient. We know this is hard for many. You may have heard the phrase, derived from a Chinese proverb, "a journey of a thousand miles begins with...a single step." Healing from pain means just taking it one step at a time. The path may meander a bit, but there is a healing path for you.

5. **This method of healing is amazing**. Be open to the wonder of it. You really can eliminate many chronic, persistent pains and other conditions by using the most complex organ in the body – the human brain – to change your body! This is now called neuroplasticity. It is remarkable and more people are experiencing this mindbody healing process in their lives.

Familiarizing Yourself with the Resources at the End of this Workbook

Before you begin your journaling, we want to remind you that we have a section at the end of this Workbook that may be useful to you during your month of writing and healing from TMS. We recommend reviewing the sections entitled "Ten Reasons You May Be Struggling to Heal" and "Ten Ways To Understand and Overcome the Issues Above." These deal with the most common issues we see for those struggling to get better. These practical tips on how to address common challenges can be useful to regularly reference in order to help you remain on your best path during the healing process.

Volume Two

We have included two versions of Day Zero based on whether or not you have first completed The MindBody Workbook (original, Vol. 1)

Day Zero if you have NOT used Volume One: Accepting the TMS Diagnosis

The first issue to focus upon is understanding and accepting the diagnosis. This day will help you look at the evidence in favor of the diagnosis and any countervailing evidence holding you back from accepting that a mindbody approach can be successful for you. We will come back to this concept weekly.

If you can make an appointment and consult with a TMS aware or expert physician, you will have had the experience of having the diagnosis confirmed. This can help you to accept the diagnosis sooner and more easily. If you have a positive or even profound initial response to reading one of the books on this subject, this can also help you accept the TMS diagnosis.

If no TMS expert is available to you, it can be helpful if another physician has reassured you that you don't need surgery or that nothing structural or biochemical clearly explains your symptoms. If an expert in his/her field directs you toward conservative treatment or non-surgical treatment, this may help you reach a mindset of accepting the TMS diagnosis.

A review with this doctor of your reports of x-rays, MRI's, and lab work may reassure you that there is nothing unusual or alarming structurally and nothing physical that clearly accounts for your symptoms.

Day Zero for you may be the day you tell your physician that you believe some or all of your condition is tension related. It may be the day that you leave your doctor's office with the recommendation to pursue a conservative program and decide to incorporate this Workbook into that conservative recommendation from your doctor. For example, a conservative approach to back pain treatment is typically a prescription for physical therapy or home exercise and anti-inflammatory or pain medication.

Goals for Day Zero are to better understand what you know and figure out what you need to learn. Also, you will want to begin gaining clarity about why the diagnosis/approach applies to you.

Day Zero if you HAVE used Volume One:
Re-Committing to TMS and Going Deeper

If you have finished *The MindBody Workbook* (original version), you are coming to this Workbook, which we call Volume Two, with some existing knowledge as well as experience in journaling. Your first step is to recommit yourself to TMS as the diagnosis that explains your symptoms. This is why you will still complete the same Day Zero Evidence Day questions. Even if your confidence is high, let yourself re-examine why TMS now makes sense as well as if there are doubts that you still need to address. Repetition is critical in order to facilitate healing and create new neural pathways!

In dealing with psychological and emotional matters, it is often necessary and beneficial to examine the same or similar issues from a slightly different vantage point or perspective. If you find that you are writing about similar feelings you've examined previously, see if you can go deeper into the feeling. Perhaps in the first 30 days of journaling you developed more of an intellectual awareness of TMS and how it applies to you, and in these 30 days you can let it sink in on a more gut and emotional level. This Workbook will also examine different areas of psychological and emotional life that will help you cover new territory.

The key for you will be to apply yourself to these 30 days of journaling with the same or greater vigor as you did for the first 30. Don't let yourself go on autopilot with your responses!

Day Zero may also involve making your first appointment with a TMS aware physician or scheduling a follow-up visit to discuss roadblocks to healing. If you have already completed *The MindBody Workbook* (Volume One) and have lingering doubts or are struggling to know how to cope with certain feelings, there is a good chance that it's time to seek professional consultation in order to bolster your confidence.

Lastly, Day Zero is a great time to make an inventory of your Type T personality characteristics and reflect on if you have been able to make changes (for example, being less hard on yourself) since you finished Volume One. If you have changed, think about how your life has improved. If you have struggled to change, re-commit to working on dialing down your Type T traits and think through what you will need to do differently.

We welcome you back on the healing journey!

Day Zero

Evidence Day

1) Why do you believe a mindbody approach makes sense in relation to your problem(s)?

___
___
___
___
___
___
___
___
___

2) Do you have some of the Type T personality characteristics listed below? How do these ways of dealing with life generate a lot of tension/stress for you?

    _____ hard on yourself
    _____ people-pleaser (sensitive to other's perceptions)
    _____ overly responsible (for everyone else?)
    _____ control-oriented
    _____ highly conscientious "goodist"
    _____ perfectionistic
    _____ worrier, often feel "uptight"

_____

_____

_____

_____

_____

_____

_____

_____

_____

_____

3) Have you suffered from other medical conditions on the list below that may be another version of a mindbody syndrome?

   ____ irritable bowel syndrome
   ____ tension headaches
   ____ unexplained pelvic pain
   ____ myofascial pain/fibromyalgia
   ____ teeth grinding
   ____ temporomandibular joint syndrome (TMJ)
   ____ medically unexplained symptoms
   ____ (other_____ specify)

   _____

   _____

   _____

   _____

   _____

   _____

   _____

   _____

   _____

4) Did your doctor's examination provide any clues that assisted her in confirming a mind-body diagnosis and excluding structural issues? If so, what?

5) What x-ray changes or laboratory findings were you informed of regarding your condition? Are any of these inconsistent, inconclusive, or benign? Do they support a mindbody diagnosis or exclude serious pathology in your case? (If this is not relevant, ask yourself: how has being informed of your test results alarmed you?)

6) On a scale of 1-10 (10 being most certain), how comfortable are you with the diagnosis of a mindbody or psychosomatic disorder? How comfortable are you with using an emotional healing approach to getting well? (Why...what is impeding you from getting to a 10?)

uncomfortable   1   2   3   4   5   6   7   8   9   10   comfortable

___

7) Is the evidence in favor of this approach enough for you? If not, what is holding you back from full acceptance? What would you need to fully accept a TMS diagnosis?

8) What have you learned about TMS/PPD so far? What do you still need to know to make you confident in moving forward?

_____

_____

_____

_____

_____

_____

9) Review the Bibliography and find an additional book that seems applicable to your problem or symptoms: For example, *Think Away Your Pain* for persistent pain, *They Can't Find Anything Wrong* for GI symptoms or medically difficult to explain symptoms, *Back in Control* for spine issues that might indicate surgery, *The MindBody Prescription* for a classic of the field that covers lots of symptoms and syndromes. Make a commitment to reading or listening (audible) to one of the above and write it down here:

_____

_____

_____

_____

_____

_____

10) New media: You may also wish to choose from the podcasts listed in Bibliography and the video links, find one that seems interesting or applicable, and listen to it in segments over the next two weeks:

___

___

___

___

___

In summary, why do you believe/accept that you have TMS?

___

___

___

___

___

___

What causes you to doubt you have TMS?

_____

_____

_____

_____

_____

_____

Day "Double Zero"

Dream Day One

Why dream when you are in pain? We find that our patients who have something to look forward to beyond their pain (TMS) often get better more quickly and feel more motivated in the face of adversity. It's often not enough to just focus on "getting rid of the pain." Focusing on moving towards your ideal life can powerfully help you get rid of pain.

1) What are some dreams you have for the future? (List and describe.)

_____

_____

_____

_____

_____

_____

_____

_____

_____

2) What is the one dream that really invigorates you when you think about it? Why this one?

_____

_____

_____

_____

_____

_____

_____

3) How did your family of origin deal with your dreams and aspirations as a child? Were you given encouragement or stifled?

_____

_____

_____

_____

_____

_____

_____

4) What steps can you take to make your dream(s) real? What is holding you back? (Again, don't let pain stop you because planning for a future is what helps the pain to go away.)

_____

_____

_____

_____

_____

_____

_____

Affirmation: I am allowed to dream.
I can pursue my dreams if I wish.

Week One

The goals of this week are to focus on accepting the diagnosis, understanding the evidence for your diagnosis, and developing confidence in this. Gradually thinking about your activity level and increasing activity is important. Beginning the march toward "thinking psychologically" will be an important phase as well.

Reading a chapter a day (or every other day) of the book(s) you selected at the end of Day Zero is an important practice. All the material you read, listen to, and review should be part of the TMS/PPD "universe." Avoid random internet searches like the plague. They can infect you with ideas and concepts that are counterproductive to your healing.

Strongly consider ending or winding down any physically-based treatments for your condition. While we advocate physical activity (and exercise) as part of your healing, we find that physical/biomechanical treatments (chiropractor, physical therapy, acupuncture, and even massage) draws the brain back to the pathways that led to the persistent pain problem.

If you've read a lot, re-reading of the material helps to "reprogram" your nervous system to heal. It takes repetition to create a habit or develop a skill (think of playing the piano). Similarly, it takes weeks (or months) of study and self-understanding to break the pattern of internalizing emotions into physical symptoms.

It takes time for emotional connections to catch up with our more rapid intellectual understanding. Intellectual acceptance of the diagnosis tends to occur first. With the work you will do, a new, deeper, more "gut" or "visceral" or "heart" level of acceptance will occur that we find is crucial for healing.

Affirmations are another tool that is extremely helpful to this process. Changing the brain and nervous system is called "neuroplasticity" and research has demonstrated that the nervous system is capable of change even into the advanced years of life. Repetition helps. We currently recommend the smartphone app **ThinkUp** because we find that it offers an easy to use, systematic way to learn from affirmations. I (Dr. Schecter) published a list of 16 Affirmations for Pain on the app (see authors/experts).

But changing your "self-talk" is even more portable than your mobile phone. Use the affirmations in this Workbook or compose your own. Positive, forward thinking messages replace the self-critical and negative internal chatter in the mind/brain that holds us back from healing and from growth. You will find affirmations throughout this workbook.

When you journal, try to express yourself spontaneously and unchecked. Do not worry about grammar or even full sentences; let it flow. By saving the journal entry, you can read and reflect on what you have written at the end of each session and more thoroughly at the end of each week. At that time, take notes and highlight phrases that are meaningful to you. Some questions will not be relevant to you; if this is the case, use the space to write about other experiences and the feelings you have. If you write particularly dark material one day and feel uncomfortable keeping it around, it is alright to tear out the page and shred or burn it if you wish. Some call this "negative" writing, but if it makes you feel safe, do it. In general, find a safe, secure space to keep your journal and you are the only one who needs to ever see or review it.

Affirmations...some more on this

Begin to develop your own "self-talk" or affirmations. These are phrases you should repeat to yourself, throughout the day, with the goal of reprogramming your nervous system through new neural pathways. They can be combined with visual images that leave you feeling peaceful and calm. Patients often choose a beach scene, sunset, mountains, music or children's faces for that sense of calmness. Ten seconds of self-talk followed by 10-15 seconds of imagery is a good combination. Repeat throughout the day as needed or as a healing habit.

An example: "I am fine, my condition is not serious, I can completely recover," or "I am healthy, my pain is from stress, and I'm learning how to deal with that."

Other Affirmations:

I can heal, I can be more active, activity is good for me.
Since my body is normal, there is nothing to fear.
Physical activity is safe and healthy for me.
I am in control—not my subconscious mind.
I learn and grow daily; my body adjusts and heals.
I think psychologically, not physically, to understand my pain.
I deal with my doubts and I accept this approach.

It can be helpful to start the day with an affirmation and each of the days that follows has one that may be helpful to you or you can write or create your own.

Week One, Day One

Emotional Landscape/Survey...

1) Do you often feel sad? (Y/N) When was the last time you felt particularly sad? Write about that experience and feeling:

_____

_____

_____

_____

_____

2) What makes you angry? Describe one or more recent or powerful anger experiences and how you felt...

_____

_____

_____

_____

_____

3) When was the last time you felt embarrassed or had a sense of shame? What did that feel like and what prompted it?

_____

_____

_____

_____

_____

4) Is there an emotion you struggle with, struggle to feel or tend to avoid feeling?

_____

_____

_____

_____

_____

Day 1. Affirmation: I am learning that my emotions are normal and that expressing my feelings is healthy.

Week One, Day Two

(Type T: Hard on Myself)

1) Do you struggle with self-criticism? What are you hard on yourself about? Talk about this a bit...

_____

_____

_____

_____

_____

2) Does your self-critical voice remind you of anyone in your life? Discuss what that was like for you and your feelings during that period?...

_____

_____

_____

_____

_____

3) When was an instance that you realized you were being too hard on yourself (e.g., another person pointed it out...)? Describe the realization and the feeling.

_____

_____

_____

_____

_____

_____

_____

Day 2. Affirmation: I am enough as I am. I am fine.

Week One, Day Three

Weekly Gratitude Journaling Day

1) What three things/people are you grateful for in your life?

_____

_____

_____

_____

_____

2) Write a paragraph about each of these things/people. Focus on the feelings they evoke and the appreciation you feel…

_____

_____

_____

_____

_____

_____

_____

Day 3. Affirmation: I appreciate what I have. I am very fortunate.

Week One, Day Four

Sadness is another important emotion

1) Describe an experience of feeling sad… what was it like? How did you cope with it? What was the root of the feeling?

_____

_____

_____

_____

_____

_____

2) How was sadness dealt with by your parents or guardians growing up?

_____

_____

_____

_____

_____

_____

3) Were you allowed to feel sad? If so, did you get comfort when you needed it? What was that like?

_____

_____

_____

_____

_____

_____

4) When was the last time you felt sad? (Expand upon the memory.)

_____

_____

_____

_____

_____

_____

Day 4. Affirmation: I accept my sadness as part of me. I grow from all my feelings and experiences.

Week One, Day Five

1) What emotion(s) are easiest for you to feel (sad, happy, angry, guilty, neutral)? What is the most common feeling you have throughout the day?

_____

_____

_____

_____

_____

2) What emotions are most difficult to access? Are there any emotions that feel scary or that you notice you actively try to avoid?

_____

_____

_____

_____

_____

3) What emotions, if any, are completely foreign to you (for example: "I never get angry")?

4) What emotions were most acceptable in your family? (Example: we had lots of anger and yelling at home, but could not talk about sadness and had to keep a stiff upper lip.)

5) What emotions were least acceptable?

___

**Day 5. Affirmation: I feel okay about my feelings.
I love myself however I feel right now.**

Week One, Day Six

1) Are there ever times where you might use emotional language, but not actually show emotion? (For example, I say that I'm sad but I'll never let myself cry.)

___

___

___

___

___

2) What were the lessons you learned about feelings growing up? (For example: "Feelings are weak" or "You aren't allowed to feel angry because you should feel grateful.")

___

___

___

___

___

3) When was the last time you felt angry? (Expand upon the memory.)

4) When was the last time you felt guilty? (Expand upon the memory.)

Day 6. Affirmation: I am resilient. I am strong.

Week One, Day Seven

Self-esteem Day

1) List three things you like about yourself (or if you struggle with this, things that others have commented upon that they like about you?)

___

___

___

___

___

2) Now write a paragraph about each of these qualities...and how you feel when you are expressing these wonderful aspects of yourself...

___

___

___

___

___

Day 7. Affirmation: I am worthwhile and valuable.

Weekly Evidence Review

Why do you believe/accept that you have TMS? Make a list.

_____

_____

_____

_____

_____

_____

What causes you to doubt it's TMS? Make a list.

_____

_____

_____

_____

_____

_____

What can you do to address doubts? List several concrete action steps you can take.

_____

_____

_____

_____

_____

_____

_____

Week Two

This week we will explore childhood and teen issues....

Week Two, Day One (Day 8)

1) Children have different "temperaments" or personalities growing up. How would you describe your personality as a child?

___

___

___

___

___

___

___

___

2) Temperaments and personalities can have more or less compatibility with other family members. How much did your personality match, or not match, with your family?

_____

_____

_____

_____

_____

_____

_____

3) Were there times growing up when you felt misunderstood? Elaborate.

_____

_____

_____

_____

_____

_____

_____

4) Were there times growing up when you had to deal with challenging experiences without support? Elaborate.

___

___

___

___

___

___

___

Day 8. Affirmation: I was totally lovable as I was...
I am totally lovable as I am today.

Week Two, Day Two (Day 9)

1) What was your family's biggest strength? How did you learn about that growing up? Did it give you strength as well?

_____

_____

_____

_____

_____

_____

2) What was your family's greatest struggle? How did you understand it as a child? How did you cope with it during that time period?

_____

_____

_____

_____

_____

_____

3) When you had a fear as a child, how would your caregivers respond?

_____

_____

_____

_____

_____

4) Did your caregivers' response make you feel better or worse? Why?

_____

_____

_____

_____

_____

**Day 9: Affirmation: I am strong. I can handle things.
I deal with my fears.**

Week Two, Day Three (Day 10)

1) What's the happiest memory you have from growing up? Write about this and how it made you feel.

___

2) What's the most difficult memory you have of growing up? How did you learn to cope with it? What feelings are evoked now thinking and writing about this?

___

3) As a child, how predictable did life feel? How much did you feel in control (or out of control)?

_____

_____

_____

_____

_____

_____

4) Were there one or more times where you felt blindsided growing up? Elaborate.

_____

_____

_____

_____

_____

_____

Day 10. Affirmation: I pride myself on learning from past mistakes.
I learn and I grow.

Week Two, Day Four (Day 11)

Gratitude Day

1) Can you think of three people or experiences you are grateful for from your childhood? List them.

___

___

___

___

___

2) Now write a paragraph about each one…take your time. If you struggle, you can go back to writing about gratitude in the present or in a period after childhood but well before today.

___

___

___

___

___

3) continue with Question 2 above

_____

_____

_____

_____

_____

_____

_____

Day 11. Affirmation: My parents and caregivers did their best. I can learn from the past and release my anger.

Week Two, Day Five (Day 12)

1) Did you have an idea growing up of what "good" children did and how they behaved? What did that mean to you then? How about now?

_____

_____

_____

_____

_____

_____

2) If you could change anything about what growing up was like, what do you wish you could change?

_____

_____

_____

_____

_____

_____

3) Were there any parts of yourself that you felt like you needed to hide growing up? Elaborate.

_____

_____

_____

_____

_____

_____

4) What did you learn about emotions growing up? Were they valued, or seen as a problem? To be expressed or to be "managed"? To be felt or ignored?

_____

_____

_____

_____

_____

_____

**Day 12. Affirmation: I am mentally and physically healthy and strong.
I can overcome.**

Week Two, Day Six (Day 13)

1) What was your caregivers' main way of showing you love and support?

_____

_____

_____

_____

_____

_____

2) How did people respond to you asking for help as a child?

_____

_____

_____

_____

_____

_____

3) How do you feel now when you ask for help? How do you feel this relates to what you learned as a child?

_____

_____

_____

_____

_____

4) Is there anything you've always wished you could communicate to your parents/caregivers? If so, elaborate.

_____

_____

_____

_____

_____

Day 13. Affirmation: I am deserving of love and support.

Week Two, Day Seven (Day 14)

Self-Esteem Day

1) List three things you liked about yourself as a teenager. If you struggle with this question, use three things that other people told you they liked about you as a child or adolescent.

_____

_____

_____

_____

_____

_____

2) Write a paragraph about each of them.

_____

_____

_____

_____

_____

_____

3) List three adolescent experiences where you felt successful, admired, or effective. Elaborate on each…

_____

_____

_____

_____

_____

_____

_____

**Day 14: Affirmation: I was once a teenager;
now I am a confident adult.**

Week Two

Childhood summary question:

If someone else had your childhood, would you think they were lucky or unlucky? Why? What would you say to that person to show you understood and to tell them they are okay?

_____

_____

_____

_____

_____

_____

_____

_____

_____

Weekly Evidence Review

In summary, why do you believe/accept that it is TMS?

_____
_____
_____
_____
_____
_____

What causes you to doubt it's TMS?

_____
_____
_____
_____
_____
_____

What can you do to erase or minimize the doubt?

___

___

___

___

___

___

Bonus Affirmation: I have learned to take care of myself and focus on my needs, as well as those of others.

Week Three

Fears/Catastrophizing/Feeling the feelings...
Identifying core fears. We know that FEAR FUELS PAIN!

Week Three, Day 1 (Day 15)

1) What are your three biggest fears at this point in your life?

___

___

___

___

___

___

___

___

___

2) Write about each of them: why do they feel so powerful to you?

___

3) Write about a time when your fears were proven wrong and how you reacted to that?

___

4) What is your style of coping with fear? (If stuck, ask yourself what you do to feel better when you are afraid or anxious.)

_____

_____

_____

_____

_____

_____

Day 15. Affirmation: I can feel fear and still make great decisions.

Week Three, Day Two (Day 16)

1) Give an example of when you assumed the worst-case scenario for a situation.

_____

_____

_____

_____

_____

_____

2) Did making this assumption lead to problems in that situation? How so?

_____

_____

_____

_____

_____

_____

3) We call this catastrophizing. Why do you think that you tend to see the cup as half empty (or three fourths) or worry that a full cup will quickly spring a leak?

_____

_____

_____

_____

_____

4) Can you give an example of when you have or how you might approach a situation from a perspective opposite of catastrophizing? (e.g. Assuming the best or believing in abundance)...

_____

_____

_____

_____

_____

Day 16. Affirmation: I can cope with difficult circumstances and successfully address problems.

Day Three, Week Three (Day 17)

Worry Day

1) List three things that make you anxious.

___

___

___

___

___

___

2) What does your anxiety feel like?

___

___

___

___

___

___

3) Does this feeling remind you of something from childhood or adolescence?

_____

_____

_____

_____

_____

4) If your friend was experiencing similar anxiety or worry, what would you tell them to help bring comfort? Can you apply this to yourself?

_____

_____

_____

_____

_____

Day 17. Affirmations: 1) I can feel calm and soothe myself.
2) My feelings are temporary; I can cope with them.

Week Three, Day Four (Day 18)

Gratitude Day

1) List three things you are thankful for this week (or in your life).

_____

_____

_____

_____

_____

_____

2) Think of one of the three above; how does it make you feel when you reflect upon that item (or person or thing)?

_____

_____

_____

_____

_____

_____

3) Feel free to write more about this item or about one of the other two things you are thankful for this week (the more detail you can use when practicing gratitude, the more grateful you will feel):

_____

_____

_____

_____

_____

_____

_____

Day 18. Affirmation: I learn to appreciate all the bounties in my life.

Week Three, Day Five (Day 19)

People with TMS often struggle with doubt, <u>including doubt about areas of life outside of TMS.</u>

1) Outside of TMS, where do you tend to experience self-doubt? When do you second-guess yourself?

___

2) Can you think of a decision in your past that you regret? How did this 'wrong' decision make you feel?

___

3) When have you taken a leap of faith in life? What helped you to go beyond your hesitation or fears and make that bold decision? If you haven't, what has stopped you?

_____

_____

_____

_____

_____

4) What would help you to feel more self-confident or trusting in your decisions? How can you get to a more decisive place?

_____

_____

_____

_____

_____

Day 19. Affirmation: I make good decisions and I learn from my mistakes. I am resilient, capable, and decisive.

Week Three, Day Six (Day 20)

Identifying your personal values can be a powerful way to strengthen your ability to commit and make values-aligned decisions.

1) What are your top 3 values in life? (Example: being a loving father; Example: acting with courage.)

_____

_____

_____

_____

_____

2) How much or how little are you acting in alignment with those values? If you are not acting in alignment with your values, what is stopping you?

_____

_____

_____

_____

_____

3) How do you deal with issues that conflict with your core values? Write about an example or two.

___

4) What would you like to commit to more fully in your life? Where would you need to take a 'leap of faith'? Is there a TMS lesson from this concept of 'commitment' and a 'leap past uncertainty'?

___

Day 20. Affirmation: I can act in accordance with my values no matter what life throws at me.

Week Three, Day Seven (Day 21)

Self-Esteem Day

1) List three things you like about yourself *right now*. (If you struggle with this, you can ask yourself what would your best friend or spouse say?)

_____

_____

_____

_____

_____

2) List three of your best life decisions. What helped you make those decisions?

_____

_____

_____

_____

_____

3) List three times in your life where you made a "mistake" but successfully recovered and learned something that helped you become stronger because of it. Write a paragraph about each.

_____

_____

_____

_____

_____

_____

_____

Day 21. Affirmation: I can feel fear, anxiety, and doubt and still live a wonderful life.

Weekly Evidence Summary

In summary, why do you believe/accept that you have TMS?

_____

_____

_____

_____

_____

_____

What causes you to doubt it's TMS?

_____

_____

_____

_____

_____

_____

What can you do this week to overcome your doubts?

Creating an Emergency Plan for Flare up of Symptoms

This week you focused on writing about anxiety and fear. One of the most common questions people have when healing from TMS is what to do when the pain significantly flares up. When dealing with a lot of pain, it becomes very difficult to think, in the moment, of what you are supposed to do, which is why knowing what to do in advance is very useful.

1) Breathing is a key element to modulating your nervous system response. Practice one minute of slow breathing focusing on the exhale. You may also want to visualize a happy or calming image while breathing.

_____

_____

_____

_____

_____

_____

_____

_____

_____

_____

2) **Self-Soothing Statement:** What can you say to yourself that is soothing? Example: I'm safe and this is just TMS. This will end.

_____

_____

_____

_____

_____

3) Remind yourself of the Top two reasons that have convinced you that you have TMS (see prior evidence sheets if needed):

_____

_____

_____

_____

_____

_____

4) What are three positive distractions you can use during a flare up?

_____

_____

_____

_____

_____

_____

5) What are three activities that help calm you down and increase your sense of emotional safety?

_____

_____

_____

_____

_____

_____

6) A Statement of Hope: what brings you hope in a moment of despair? For example: I have read about so many people healing from challenging TMS symptoms. I can heal, too! Or, I have gotten better before using this approach, it can work again!

___

___

___

___

___

___

___

We recommend taking your answers from the above and creating an "Emergency Pain Note" in your phone. This note is something that you can refer to when you are having a flare up that can calm you and offer reassurance. It is a quick reference when your mind is not in the best condition to think through how to handle the flareup.

Week Four

Week Four, Day One (Day 22)

Self Compassion, Self Care and Play

This week we will focus on an area of life often neglected and very important for healing and for ongoing flourishing!

1) Sometimes people believe self-criticism helps them succeed or do well in life. What are the pros and cons of being highly self-critical?

___
___
___
___
___
___
___

2) Describe an incident(s) when you have been highly self-critical in your life. How did you feel about this and how did you or might you get out of this cycle?

3) What are the benefits of being self-compassionate, self-nurturing or self-soothing? Have you had any experiences with this to discuss?

4) Can you see a connection between your approach to criticism and self-compassion and how it relates to your childhood experience? Please elaborate.

Day 22. Affirmation: I can be kind to myself, self-loving, and still be successful.

Week Four, Day Two (Day 23)

1) Self-criticism and criticism of others are highly associated with each other. Identify three people or situations in which you can be more kind and compassionate.

_____

_____

_____

_____

_____

2) In what ways are you self-critical in relation to TMS healing? (Example: beating yourself up for not having healed quickly enough.)

_____

_____

_____

_____

_____

3) Do you hold constantly high expectations for yourself? Elaborate. Is this innate to you or reflecting your upbringing? Or both?

_____

_____

_____

_____

_____

_____

4) What feelings, thoughts, or parts of yourself are you most critical of? How might you be kinder to yourself about these issues?

_____

_____

_____

_____

_____

_____

Day 23. Affirmation: I am courageous for committing to heal from TMS.

Week Four, Day Three (Day 24)

Play has positive effects on the nervous system, reduces worry, and calms us down. Today's writing is focused on examining your relationship with play.

1) Growing up, what did you enjoy doing for play? How did you feel while doing this?

_____

_____

_____

_____

_____

2) How playful is your life currently? What do you do now to play?

_____

_____

_____

_____

_____

3) What is one activity you would enjoy doing if you had more time? What is getting in the way of making time for play? (We know you're busy.)

___

4) How will you integrate play into your weekly schedule? Things that are not scheduled often do not get done. Can you make this a priority? If not, why?

___

Day 24. Affirmation: I deserve to play.
I prioritize my enjoyment of life.

Week Four, Day Four (Day 25)

Gratitude Day

1) Describe a recent experience in which you felt cared for or helped by an unexpected person.

_____

_____

_____

_____

_____

_____

2) Who is someone that has offered you protection, guidance, or wisdom in your life?

_____

_____

_____

_____

_____

_____

3) List three people this week that you appreciate. Can you go forward and actually say thank you to them? How do you feel in response?

_____

_____

_____

_____

_____

4) List three people who are either deceased or you are no longer in contact with, and write a brief thank you letter to each of them.

_____

_____

_____

_____

_____

Day 25. Affirmation: I am thankful for those that have contributed to my growth and well-being.

Week Four, Day Five (Day 26)

1) Describe a recent situation in which you were especially hard on yourself. Include up to three self-critical thoughts you had about yourself.

_____

_____

_____

_____

_____

2) If a friend was in the same situation, list three considerate responses or compassionate statements you would offer them.

_____

_____

_____

_____

_____

3) What statements of compassion do you need to offer yourself more frequently?

4) What could be holding you back from this? Think back to childhood experiences, parents, supervisors, professors, etc.

Day 26. Affirmation: I speak gently to myself with words of encouragement that I would also share with others.

Week Four, Day Six (Day 27)

We sometimes feel uncomfortable saying or thinking that we deserve certain things in life (especially in respect to relationships, work, and health). Most of these important ones are non-material.

1) What three things do you really deserve? (E.g., a positive relationship, a better job, better health, a sense of purpose.)

___

___

___

___

___

2) Does it feel uncomfortable writing about 'deserving' things? Why so?

___

___

___

___

___

___

___

3) Growing up, did you feel deserving of good things happening to you? Why or why not?

4) Are you comfortable with believing and saying that you deserve to be pain free? Elaborate.

Day 27. Affirmation: I deserve to be pain free!

Week Four, Day Seven (Day 28)

Self-Esteem day

1) What do you like about yourself this week? Perhaps your courage to answer the questions posed honestly and openly?

_____

_____

_____

_____

_____

2) What are you most proud of in your life?

_____

_____

_____

_____

_____

3) What is something in your life now that makes you feel highly effective?

_____

_____

_____

_____

_____

_____

4) What are you proud of in your TMS journey so far?

_____

_____

_____

_____

_____

_____

**Day 28. Affirmation: I am a strong person.
I take on challenges and succeed.**

Final Days

Day 29

Dream Day Two

We find that our patients who have something to look forward to beyond their pain (TMS) often get better more quickly. Focusing on moving towards your ideal life can powerfully help you get rid of pain.

1) Have you thought more about your dream(s) from the first Dream Day and have you taken any actions? Elaborate.

_____

_____

_____

_____

_____

_____

_____

2) What is the one dream that really invigorates you when you think about it? Why this one?

3) How do people in your life currently deal with your dreams and aspirations? Do you feel supported and encouraged, or do they treat you like your dreams are silly?

4) What steps can you take to make your dream(s) real? What is holding you back? (Again, don't let pain stop you, because planning for a future is what helps pain to go away.)

___

___

___

___

___

___

___

Day 29. Affirmation: I am allowed to dream.
I can pursue my dreams if I wish.
My dreams can be unlimited.

Day 30

Reflection Day

1) What are the three biggest lessons you've learned from journaling in this workbook for a month?

___

___

___

___

___

___

2) What will be your action steps after you complete this workbook?

___

___

___

___

___

___

3) What feeling or life issue will need more attention from you going forward?

_____

_____

_____

_____

_____

4) What part of your life (play, friends, work, etc.) needs some reconfiguring based upon your writing this month?

_____

_____

_____

_____

_____

Day 30. Affirmation: I continue to learn.
I enjoy becoming more aware.
I am healing my mind and body.

Affirmations

Further Use

Pick three affirmations from the last 30 days that are meaningful to you and write them on post-its. Repeat them frequently and keep them on your mirror if you can. You can list their locations below and write them out as well.

page _____

page _____

page _____

_____

_____

_____

_____

_____

_____

The MindBody Workbook Volume Two

Final Evidence Summary

In summary, why do you believe/accept that it is TMS?

_____

_____

_____

_____

_____

What causes you to doubt it's TMS?

_____

_____

_____

_____

_____

What is left to wipe away the doubts? (Also see the Afterword section.)

Afterword and Appendices

So you've finished the *MindBody Workbook, Volume Two* (and maybe Volume One, as well). Congratulations are in order. It takes real courage to heal.

What's next? First, assess where you are with your health. If you have made substantial progress, this certainly speaks to the efficacy of the mindbody approach with your disorder. The progress you've made should build upon itself and continue to grow. You can come back and reread your entries at any time, approaching them with a fresh perspective. You may even decide to continue keeping a journal, or even answering these questions a second time in a blank notebook.

People often ask what to journal about next. A simple formula for your daily journaling entries is to write about *what happened that day, what you thought about, and what you felt.* Type-T personalities can sometimes worry if they are journaling "right." You don't need to worry about this too much. The main goal is to keep in touch with your emotions and continue to regularly express yourself. The best journaling session is the one that you have! You can also use the original *MindBody Workbook* as a vehicle for another 30 days of journaling.

If you've made little or no progress with your condition, or gotten worse, it's time to reassess the situation (see our Top 10 List below for further ideas). If you haven't already, it is time for you to be seen by a qualified physician, preferably mindbody-oriented. This might be a reexamination or perhaps a first visit. If the doctor finds nothing of concern, or no change in his original assessment, then you've got more work to do. You're an excellent candidate for a mindbody psychotherapist in your area. Most importantly, stay positive and practice self-kindness. It takes people different amounts of time to heal and just because it might take you longer does not mean you are a failure at this approach.

If you are still having a great deal of difficulty accepting your condition as psychophysiologic or believing in the power of the mindbody connection, then reading or rereading one of the books in the bibliography pertinent to this subject is appropriate. Dealing with your doubt intellectually and also dealing with the emotional issues underlying your doubt is crucial. A good psychotherapist can be crucial to elucidating these factors.

Breaking the cycle of pain takes some people a short time and others somewhat longer. If you are in the latter category, don't despair. Taking longer to improve does not mean you won't be successful with this approach in the longer run. While your path may be different, your commitment to look inside yourself for answers, and complete this thirty day program, speaks forcefully to your ultimate success. Keep going...

If you find that you are having a hard time healing and have a lot of questions about how to go about your healing program, we also recommend our online video course called *The MindBody Healing Journey*. Consisting of five hours of videos in shorter segments, including a substantial section that answers the most commonly asked questions that we have addressed in our clinical practices, and downloadable documents (pdf's), it offers a detailed, comprehensive, but concise approach to understanding and relieving chronic pain. Many have described it as a calming influence as well. https://www.mindbodymedicine.com/online-course

U.S. and International Therapists and Physicians are listed on Dr. Schechter's website:

Doctors: https://www.mindbodymedicine.com/doctors-page
Therapists: https://www.mindbodymedicine.com/therapists-links

Ten Reasons You May Be Struggling to Heal

If you find that you are having a hard time healing and aren't sure why, here are 10 common issues we've seen:

1) Doubt is a crippler – You are still stuck on a previous structural explanation you received for your pain.
2) Over-intellectualizing: You have accepted the diagnosis in your head, but not in your heart.
3) Commitment: You've struggled to take the full "leap of faith" with your healing and have engaged with your healing program only partially.
4) Emotional "repression": Even though you've tried to access your emotions, it's continued to be a substantial challenge.
5) Overactivation of fight/flight: Your stress levels have remained consistently high to the point that it's been hard to calm down.
6) Go Deeper: You have identified emotional issues, but there are deeper inner conflicts that you have struggled to address.
7) Overdoing it: You have become obsessed with healing but actually need to focus on resuming what brings you joy in life (see your dream day entries).
8) Fear of permanence: You have not accepted that this pain can and will go away!
9) Fear of movement: You're afraid to hurt yourself, have a flareup or don't trust your body to exercise.
10) Fear fuels the pain: The fear of the pain is so great that it's been hard to do the necessary emotional work.

Ten Ways To Understand and Overcome the Issues Above

1) Doubt: Go see a TMS medical provider. Get a diagnosis! Have someone obtain and review imaging if that would reassure you.
2) Intellectualizing: Do less reading and thinking and focus on expressing your feelings. Ask yourself what is the evidence you would need to emotionally accept you have TMS? Also consider if you are overly skeptical in general and if so address this tendency.
3) Commitment: What is holding you back? Take the 'leap'. Or analyze what is the impediment?
4) Repression: Determine what makes it hard to feel. Is it a lack of feeling safe enough to 'let it out?' Is there a fear that you might feel too much? Or become overwhelmed? If you are stuck, either talk with a friend, loved one, or therapist to help get past the emotional block.
5) Fight/flight: Vacation, meditation, breathing, reduce life stress. Sometimes, but certainly not always, healing from TMS involves real life changes, not just acknowledgment of feelings and just changing your thoughts!
6) Depth: Meet with a therapist with a more psychodynamic or analytic style.
7) Overdoing/obsessing about healing: Limit yourself to 30 minutes every other day of TMS "work" and add back more time to play.
8) Fear of permanence: Most people don't live with pain their whole lives. Why should you be the one? Are you stuck in a loop, catastrophizing? Can you move forward from that?
9) Fear of movement: Start slowly, walk, move, build up gradually.
10) Fear of pain: Where is this coming from? TMS is real pain, but not damage. What can help you to calm down even when you're in discomfort?

Finding a MindBody Practitioner

We use the term mindbody throughout this workbook. However, a mindbody doctor is hard to find and harder to classify. Many primary care physicians have a holistic emphasis. An individual trained in pain management may combine up to date physical and imaging skills along with a psychological mindset.

Doctors who have trained with or been cured by the work of Dr. John Sarno may be a good place to start in looking for a mindbody cure. At this time, there are a few dozen of these individuals nationally or internationally. Many are mentioned on the web site www.mindbodymedicine.com. Others are listed on the www.PPDassociation.org website. The ability to be knowledgeable in the conventional diagnosis or treatment of a condition is important, as well as the specialized knowledge of TMS diagnosis and its treatment.

Ideally, a mindbody practitioner should be psychologically aware of him/herself. He may have a background or exposure to psychology or psychiatric diagnosis. This mindbody approach is, in the truest sense, holistic. It is alternative only in the sense that mainstream medicine is not biopsychosocial in outlook. Much of the mainstream is very reductionistic and biomedical exclusively.

If a TMS practitioner is not available in your area, consider a telemedicine visit with one. Get imaging or lab testing first and send that to the doctor. If your psychosomatic problem is not back pain, find a doctor who specializes in that problem or a good primary care physician. Preferably, look for an open-minded, empathic individual open to psychological aspects of illness. Unfortunately, this is not that simple. If all else fails, settle with someone with good technical training and expertise who can exclude serious pathology (cancer, fractures, infection, etc.).

Ask the doctor if a conservative program is suitable. If he agrees, begin the mindbody program, along with other treatments he may recommend. If the doctor advises surgery, get a second opinion in your area. If necessary, get a third opinion. Some conditions require surgery—be sure to have the best surgeon you can find and get the least surgery that can treat the condition effectively. If the doctor agrees, a purely psychological program of devoting yourself to the Workbook for thirty days and deferring other treatments is often most effective. However, the Workbook can certainly be combined with other treatments that alleviate pain, increase flexibility, and improve strength. It's also worth noting that even if you need surgery, research suggests that the outcome will be better if you are less stressed and in a better place emotionally.

Common sense should prevail. Your local doctor is your medical advisor. If what he says makes sense to you, then follow it wholeheartedly. If you're not getting better, seek other opinions. A good primary care doctor who specializes in family practice or internal medicine is often the best person with whom to talk about holistic medicine. They can also be your advocate or interpreter of specialist's recommendations for your care. Finally, they are usually the best judges of whether your psychological status requires psychotherapy, antidepressant medications, anti-anxiety medications, or a combination of these.

Psychiatrists and psychologists often suffer from the same mind/body split as the rest of the medical field. Try to find one who is familiar with TMS, open to reading the book, or adept with psychosomatic disorders. At a minimum, your therapist should believe that the mind and emotions influence the body. Explain to them that you don't want to learn how to cope with the pain, you want to understand how your emotions may be causing or contributing to it. If they are not open to this concept, seek out another therapist. You can also find a list of mind-body therapists at https://ppdassociation.org/directory

You are in charge of whom you see and what treatments you accept. They are there to advise and care for you.

Bonus: Other Approaches to Journaling

After this Workbook, you may be interested in continuing to journal and want to explore different journaling approaches. Journaling is writing about thoughts and feelings. These include things we feel today and things we have felt for a long time. When done effectively, the focus is not grammar or logic, it is expression and association.

The term "free association" refers to connections that we spontaneously make between our feelings today and past experiences. These past events may be in childhood, teen years or adulthood. Be open to the power of your psychological memories, especially from your youth.

How is this different from "dear diary"? Journaling is purposeful. It is not about what we did today, it is about what we thought about and how we felt. By having guidance, like through this Workbook, one can systematically work through the different important parts of life and look for the emotional stressors and powerful feelings that underlie our daily life. Work life, love life, financial issues, children, parents, school, and other areas of life are covered in the Workbook and are highly important to write about.

One of the basic questions in Journaling is "What's going on in my life?" You can always fall back on this. But more specifically, what makes you angry? What makes you sad? What makes you anxious? Start the writing and the feelings and thoughts and connections will flow. Like any activity, you improve with practice, with effort, and with time. Be patient, but persistent.

While journaling requires some time and some effort, it is worth it because the results can be powerful and amazing. This type of guided journaling can also be referred back to at a later date which is the value of keeping your writing. On the other hand, if you feel safer destroying what you wrote or if you enjoy the catharsis of getting rid of the pages, then feel free to do that instead.

There are quite a few ways to journal or do expressive writing. You may wish to try other types to see what works for you. Here are some examples:

1) <u>Guided journaling</u> is the focus of this Workbook. We provide you with prompts and you focus your attention on answering these prompts. Note that you are not restricted to only writing an answer, but also encouraged to make associations and connections between the present and the past and between last week's writing and today's where possible.

2) <u>Stream of consciousness</u> writing at its purest is literally putting pen to paper and writing down whatever one thinks of and continuing this for an interval of time. Some people use an hourglass sand timer or a phone timer for five or ten minutes for this purpose. This is an extreme form of *don't edit and don't restrict what you write down*. Sometimes it might be gibberish because the brain generates a lot of random thoughts.

3) <u>In cathartic writing</u>, also known as dark writing, the goal is to write as darkly as possible, tapping into anger and other harsh, painful, and ugly or uncomfortable feelings. Some describe this as akin to a written, waking nightmare. Most people who do dark writing do it for a few days at a time or even less often. This writing is often reviewed and then torn up, shredded, or even burnt as part of the catharsis.

4) <u>Reflective writing</u> involves reflecting and writing about a topic or a thought or a theme and free writing about that. DS sometimes picks a topic or two for a patient in the office and suggests they make that the subject of their writing for a day or two. Some individuals are great at finding topics on their own. These might include: my job; my career future; my relationship with mom; my boss; my ex-girlfriend.

Good luck.

Bibliography

Back Pain, TMS

Sarno, J., *Healing Back Pain*, Warner Books, New York, 1991.
Sarno, J., *The MindBody Prescription*, Warner Books, New York, 1998.
Schechter, D. *The MindBody Workbook (original)*, MindBody Medicine Publications, LA, 1999.
Schechter, D. *Think Away Your Pain*, MindBody Medicine Publications. LA. 2014
Hanscom, D. *Back in Control*, Vertus Press. Seattle. 2012
Schubiner, H. *Unlearn Your Pain*, Mind Body Publishing, LLC, 2022.
Clarke, Schechter, Schubiner. *Diagnostic Guide to Psychophysiologic Disorders*, 2022

Mind-Body Connection

Van der Kolk, Bessel. *The Body Keeps the Score*, Penguin, 2015.
Gabor Mate, *When the Body Says No*, Wiley. 2011.
Ozanich, Steven. *The Great Pain Deception*. 2011.

Psychology of TMS

Gordon, A and Ziv, A. *The Way Out*, Avery, 2022.
Anderson, F. and Sherman, E. *Pathways to Pain Relief*. 2013.

Self Compassion/Positive Psychology

Neff, Kristin. *The Self-Compassion Workbook*. Guilford Press, 2018
Lyubomirsky, S. *The How of Happiness*. Penguin, 2007.

About the Authors

David Schechter, MD is a board-certified family medicine/sports medicine physician and a credentialed pain practitioner who has explored the mindbody connection in his medical training, clinical practice and research for over thirty years. Inspired by the writings of George Engel, MD about the biopsychosocial model of disease and the pioneering work of John Sarno, MD on Tension Myoneural Syndrome, he has incorporated an integrated mindbody approach into his unique clinical practice.

Over the last twenty seven years, Dr. Schechter has further focused on the treatment of back pain, neck pain, RSI and other disorders, using a mindbody approach. The essence has been to teach patients not to fear their pain and to heal by acknowledging and connecting the pain to the underlying emotional issues in their lives. Dr.Schechter has helped many thousands of patients from all over the United States, from Canada, Mexico, Europe, and Asia.

Dr. Schechter has had an academic appointment at the USC School of Medicine and has taught medical students and residents. He has lectured at medical conferences and meetings. In addition to this Workbook, and the original MindBody Workbook, he is the author of **Think Away Your Pain** (2014) which offers clear, user-friendly explanations, more treatment focus, and more. He has produced an audio program/mp3 (The MindBody AudioProgram) and a DVD (The MindBody Patient Panel). For information, free podcasts, or to order items, go to www.MindBodyMedicine.com. For practice information and forms, review www.SchechterMD.com.

Dr. Schechter lives in Los Angeles with his wife; two sons are in and out. His office is located in Culver City. Dr. Schechter was the Principal Investigator of the Seligman Medical Institute and he published research on this topic: www.mindbodymedicine.com/research-smi

There are also videos on a "you tube channel" that include patient testimonials and brief discussions of the condition and its treatment by Dr. Schechter. http://www.youtube.com/user/mindbodydr Dr. Schechter's facebook page is www.facebook.com/DSMDCulverCity On twitter, @pain_md_la

Justin Barker, Psy.D. is a Clinical Psychologist who received his doctorate from the Rutgers Graduate School of Applied and Professional Psychology. After successfully healing from chronic back pain with a TMS approach, Dr. Barker focused his dissertation research on examining a new method of combining TMS theory with psychotherapy treatment. After practicing in Los Angeles for a few years, he reached out to Dr. Schechter to explore collaborative opportunities in TMS treatment.

During the COVID-19 pandemic, Dr. Schechter and Dr. Barker designed and established an online Zoom group for TMS patients called the TMS Healing Group. The group has been a space for patients to come together and learn from each other and us about how to heal as well as address common challenges in healing. Both Dr. Schechter and Dr. Barker share the belief that combining medical and psychological expertise represents a powerful combination to facilitate healing.

As the TMS Healing Group continued to grow and be refined it became increasingly clear that as TMS information has proliferated, so has confusion about the "right" approach or the necessary steps to healing. This was the catalyst for the Online Course, *The MindBody Healing Journey*, a comprehensive detailed video program (with pdf's) that guides a patient through the stages of healing from chronic pain and other mind-body symptoms. Dr. Barker and Dr. Schechter's hope with the course was to create a clear, straightforward, calming, and manageable path to healing in a concise format.

As Dr. Schechter and Dr. Barker continued to collaborate and develop a shared language for TMS healing, Dr. Schechter invited Dr. Barker to help create the Second Volume of the MindBody workbook.

Dr. Barker is in private practice with mostly virtual psychotherapy clients. In addition to treating TMS, he specializes in anxiety disorders, obsessive-compulsive disorder, and trauma. www.drjustinbarker.com

Dr. Barker lives near the beach in Los Angeles with his wife. Outside of the therapy office, he enjoys spending time on the sand, cooking, going to the theater, museums, spending time with friends and family and anything else that provides the sense of play so important for Type-T personalities.

The MindBody Healing Journey

Praise for the online course:

From Patients:

"Whether you are initially exploring if TMS/Mind-Body is the cause of your symptoms or are in the final stages of recovery, this course is the most comprehensive material I have found! It explores both the medical issues and psychological causes. Dr. Schechter walks you through the initial diagnosis and explains how to apply the treatment approach. Dr. Barker explains the typical psychological causes and how to improve in those areas applicable to you. Both Doctors then answer many questions.

This program of treatment has been successful for me. I used to be on high dose opioids and a spinal cord stimulator. I have tapered off the opioids and the stimulator is turned off. It works!"

Jim H., Patient. Southern California

"The course was fabulous! It is so helpful to have so much information and advice (and current information) in one place, in a format that is easy for even someone in severe pain to access. I have previously found TMS information to be a lot of work to piece together. This course is much needed.

I found the course to be comprehensive and clear. It answered most of the questions that had been lingering ... I particularly appreciated the very comprehensive FAQ sections and the PDF list of question topics, which made it easy to find answers to the most personally relevant questions before listening to the full recording."

Jen. M., Patient Santa Barbara, CA

"Thank you both for your compassionate and comprehensive approach to helping TMS sufferers to become more aware of how the brain and emotions are at play in our physical pain. It's been 5 years now since my debilitating symptoms began... Your course has added a new dimension in education to the cause of recovery from this syndrome. Much appreciated!"

L. Campbell, Ontario, CAN

"My favorite part was the FAQ. I feel like it answered many questions that contributed to doubts I had and it would do the same for other patients..."

P.T., Patient, Los Angeles

"Dear Dr. Schechter. I just want to say how much I like listening to Dr. Barker. He gives so much information that I can relate to, at a nice easy pace, and with a very kind demeanor. Your program is awesome. Thank you."

Albert N, Patient, Los Angeles

From Professionals:

"The course did a great job of explaining TMS in a way that is easily understandable and relatable. The MBHJ course truly reflects a well-rounded, patient-centered care approach. It is an affordable investment for those with chronic pain and TMS to learn how to take a more effective and holistic approach to solve their pain problem. By the end of the course, TMS patients can see life in a new light that helps them heal from emotional build-up, interact with themselves more empathetically, set healthy boundaries, and grow as a whole person."

Amari Dior, TMS Pain and Life coach

"This course is comprehensive, profound, and empowering. Dr. Schechter and Dr. Barker have done a wonderful job explaining evidence-based mind-body healing modalities, intricate emotional patterns contributing to pain, and addressing common questions and challenges from their years of experience treating patients with TMS. This course might be a game-changer for patients looking for answers to their chronic pain!"

Priyanka Chitti M.B.B.S, Medical Doctor

"Dr. Schechter (MD) and Dr. Barker (Psychologist) provide a beautiful pairing of professions to amplify, and highlight, the holistic approach to TMS/MindBody Syndrome. This course was thoughtfully structured, as a guide, to help patients understand and work through their TMS/PPD issues."

Vanessa Sedano, ACSW, Los Angeles

"Dr. Schechter and Dr. Barker are veterans in the field of mind-body medicine, and this program they've put together provides a concise education on TMS and the recovery process. They provide simple, yet powerful tools to use on one's Healing Journey in a format that is very user friendly and easy to navigate"

Daniel Gaines, LCSW

Other Books by David Schechter, M.D.

The MindBody Workbook (original version)
Think Away Your Pain
Understanding and Healing From TMS (derived from an older Audio Program)

Made in the USA
Las Vegas, NV
21 September 2024